THE SMOKING EPIDEMIC

A prescri
change

CW01046437

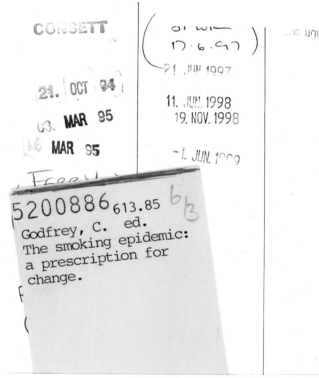

DURHAM COUNTY COUNCIL
Arts, Libraries and Museums Department

Please return or renew this item by the last date shown.
Fines will be charged if the book is kept after this date.
Thank you for using *your* library.

100% recycled paper

Report written by
Christine Godfrey
Martin Raw
Matthew Sutton
Hilly Edwards

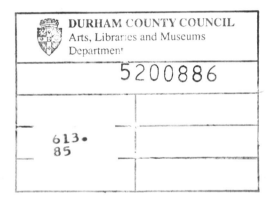

The HEA is grateful to the Office of Population Censuses and Surveys
for permission to use data from the 1988 and the 1990 General
Household Survey.

ISBN 1 85448 964 X

Health Education Authority
Hamilton House
Mabledon Place
London WC1H 9TX

Typesetting by Type Generation
Printed in Great Britain by The KPC Group, London and Ashford, Kent

CONTENTS

ACKNOWLEDGEMENTS

There are many people who need thanking as this project was truly a concerted team effort. Christine Godfrey and Martin Raw are particularly appreciated for their determination and humour. Matthew Sutton and Hilly Edwards, both highly motivated and quietly competent, worked hard in order to achieve extremely tight deadlines.

Special thanks to Julia Wadsworth and Debbie Forrest, both of whom work in primary care. They attended meetings, read drafts, found ex-smokers to talk to us, and generally contributed creative ideas and support to all aspects of the project. Adrian Roxan, of the BMA Public Affairs Division, brought to bear his usual bright perceptive wit and gave invaluable advice on the role of GPs in reducing the number of smokers.

Many others have helped in many ways, especially by discussing the project with us, correcting our misperceptions about primary care and reading and criticising drafts: Penny Astrop, Helen Charley, Andy Haines, Sarah Hall, Alanah Houston, David Raw. Kevin McConway gave indispensable assistance making sure our Macs and PCs could talk to each other, and Jean Morgan with typing. Particular thanks are also due to Professor Nick Bosanquet for his expert advice and input.

As usual, colleagues from the HEA, the HEA Helios project, the HEA Primary Health Care Unit, and Health Promotion Wales gave their own inimitable brand of expertise and support: Bill Bellew, Cecilia Farren, Elaine Fulard, John Griffiths, Sonya King, Dee McLean, Fran Nelson, Judith Watt, and Kate Woodhouse.

We would also like to thank the ex-smokers who were prepared to talk to us, some of whose words are used in this report.

Katie Aston
Project Manager
October 1993

FOREWORD

The Smoking Epidemic: A prescription for change is the third report in a series focusing attention on the costs of smoking to individuals and to the health service. It describes the costs of smoking to the primary health care system in England and Wales. Such costs have not been shown before in a systematic way. By comparing smokers and non-smokers the report shows that smoking accounts for an additional eight million GP consultations per year and over seven million prescriptions per year at a total cost of well over £140 million. Including the estimated costs to the NHS of outpatient and inpatient services resulting from these GP consultations the total annual cost is over £610 million.

This report emphasises not only the considerable costs of smoking to the primary health care system, but the crucial role of the primary health care team in reducing smoking prevalence. They occupy a strategic position because so many people come into contact with them. Across the UK, about 250,000 smokers visit their GP every day. Their potential impact is therefore enormous. The evidence quoted in this report is that the practice team can be effective in helping smokers to stop.

The previous reports in this series are *The Smoking Epidemic: Counting the cost*, launched in November 1991, which detailed the costs of smoking to health authorities and to local government districts, providing reliable and up to date estimates of the damaging effects of tobacco. *The Smoking Epidemic: A manifesto for action*, launched in 1992, which presented similar data for UK and European parliamentary constituencies and, for the first time, showed how many people are exposed to passive smoking in their homes through living with smokers.

Both reports gave estimates of the overall effects of smoking. In the UK some 111,000 premature deaths a year are caused by smoking – about 300 deaths a day or one every five minutes! Hospital admissions due to illness from smoking number 284,000 each year, occupying an average of 9,500 hospital beds every day and at an annual cost to the NHS of over £400 million – more than £1,000,000 a day or £600 a minute. These statistics emphasise that smoking continues to cost the country dearly and that action to prevent this massive burden of destruction remains urgently needed.

There are many actions that GPs and the whole of the primary health care team can take to contribute to the smoking targets contained in *The Health of the Nation*, in particular to reduce the prevalence of cigarette smoking to no more than 20 per cent by the year 2000 in both men and women aged 16 and over.

The British public consider advice from a GP as the most trustworthy source available. After receiving advice from a GP opportunistically during a routine consultation, six out of ten British smokers try to stop, and up to five per cent of all those so advised may succeed. There is, however, ample scope for increased activity; in 1983 only 22 per cent of British smokers reported having ever received advice from a GP to stop smoking; a further 11 per cent had been urged to cut down. These figures were virtually unchanged in 1990, at 26 per cent and 7 per cent respectively, resulting in a huge lost opportunity to help people live healthier lives. About 70 per cent of English adults, and therefore about 8 million smokers, see their doctor each year. Up to 5 per cent of these, or 400,000 smokers, might give up each year if advised regularly to stop. In addition GPs and the primary health care team can invest in the health of future generations by talking to parents about the strong influence that their smoking has on whether their children start to smoke. By supporting smokers to stop, GPs can also protect the health of the one-half of all children in the UK who are exposed to tobacco smoke at home.

Furthermore, as respected members of their communities, GPs have great influence, far greater on MPs for example than any other professional group, and can add weight to local campaigns such as No Smoking Day by speaking to the public though the local media. Media and publicity about smoking are particularly important in influencing public opinion, and bringing about changes in public policies in favour of all the measures necessary to achieve the Health of the Nation targets.

Dr Spencer Hagard
Chief Executive
Health Education Authority

PROLOGUE

This report emphasises just how much smoking costs us in primary care and reminds us of the importance of encouraging smokers to stop. In the long term the potential savings of our time and resources are enormous and reinforce the emphasis on smoking cessation in *The Health of the Nation*. Perhaps more important, the initial time investment in advising smokers to stop would be repaid by the improvements to their health. As a GP who believes in prevention I welcome this report and urge my colleagues to adopt the guidelines provided in Chapter 3.

Margaret Safranek
General practitioner

In general practice we are in an ideal position to provide support and encouragement when our patients are ready to stop. By repeatedly giving a consistent message, we can have a cumulative effect over the years. In my work with asthma patients, the smoking habit tends to cloud the existing disease, and it is only once smokers have stopped that we can effectively deal with their symptoms. This report emphasises that by helping our patients to stop, we will eventually free time to concentrate on their chronic problems.

Suzanne Brooks
Practice nurse

This report should provide tremendous encouragement to all those working in general practice, from the GP to the practice nurse, to the staff who keep the leaflet rack stocked. It makes clear why smoking cessation is so important and gives welcome practical advice on what to do. Once we believe that, by helping smokers to stop, general practice can have a significant impact on the health of our patients, I trust we will all be motivated to do more in this vital area.

Julia Wadsworth
Practice manager

INTRODUCTION

Smoking-related diseases account for a significant use of professionals' time in primary care. Smoking impairs the health and finances of smokers. It is the largest single cause of preventable and premature death, causing 111 000 deaths a year in the UK in 1991.[1]

This report shows:

- how smoking-related diseases affect the work of the primary care team
- how the primary care team can help smokers stop
- that the primary care team can be effective in helping smokers stop.

Many smokers want to stop smoking, and primary health care professionals can help them do so using a simple approach outlined in Chapter 3 of this report. By doing so, they can:

- save time and resources spent on treating smoking-related diseases in the long term
- reduce the incidence of smoking-related diseases and deaths
- reduce the effects of passive smoking
- improve the health of patients and their families
- increase job satisfaction by providing effective help in stopping.

Background to this report

This report follows others which gave reliable estimates of the damaging effects of smoking on the nation's health and costs to NHS hospitals. In 1985 *The Big Kill* showed the effects of smoking on NHS and local authority districts, and Westminster and European parliamentary constituencies in England and Wales.[2] In 1991 *The Smoking Epidemic: Counting the Cost* updated the information on smoking-related deaths, hospital use and costs for each health region, health district, and local authority district.[1] And in 1992 *The Smoking Epidemic: a Manifesto for Action* provided similar figures for UK and European parliamentary constituencies.[3]

The government white paper *The Health of the Nation* in 1992 set targets for health which include reducing smoking by one-third.[4] Interventions by primary health care teams can make a significant contribution to meeting this target.

The costs of smoking to primary care

Compared with non-smokers, smokers:

- see their GP more often
- have more prescriptions
- are more likely to be referred to hospital for an outpatient appointment.

The main resource in primary care is professionals' time. Sicker patients require more time. Smoking affects smokers *and* their families, particularly children. Despite a fall in the numbers of adults who smoke, over 30 per cent of the adult population still smokes and 51 per cent of children live in a household in which at least one person smokes. Children express concern about their parents' smoking as shown by this quote from a parent: *But as the children have got older they come home with different remarks, passive smoking especially, smell of cigarette smoke and it got to 'you're killing yourself' and 'we want you to be here for a long time'.* General practitioners are usually the first point of contact to the health services for any illness. Primary health care teams provide care for people with chronic smoking-related diseases such as cancer, heart disease or stroke.

Stopping smoking at almost any age improves health, although the earlier people stop the greater the health gain and potential cost savings, and obviously best of all would be if people never started in the first place. The benefits can be marked as this ex-smoker testifies: *Well, I'm just as normal as the next person now, and it's all because I've stopped smoking. I'm swimming with the children now, play football, want to do more things because I've got more time, whereas before I used to want to just sit down and have a cigarette and a cup of coffee. I could only swim a width and I'd be out of breath, and I'd think. 'Oh God no, I've got to get out and have a cigarette!' Once you turn to the other side you really go the whole hog. The children, the house,* everything *is a lot better, and my husband is a lot happier. I hope I've given the children the example at the right time.* Onset of a smoking-related disease often motivates smokers to stop. Commitment to helping smokers stop needs to be a permanent feature of primary care.

This report shows the costs of smoking in primary care. It does not attempt to calculate the human misery resulting from the effects of smoking, nor the advantages to ex-smokers who have given up. However we have illustrated the key themes of this report with quotes from ex-smokers who talked to us about their smoking and the benefits of giving up. They are from London and the Midlands.

Estimating the costs to primary care

These costs have been estimated by comparing the use of health services by smokers and non-smokers. Data from the General Household Survey were used to calculate:

- time for smokers' additional consultations due to smoking-related illnesses
- resource costs of these consultations
- cost of additional prescriptions
- estimated costs of outpatient and inpatient hospital visits arising from the additional visits to the GPs.

Smoking rates vary across the country and between GP practices. Typical profiles are constructed for a typical GP, a rural GP and an urban GP for each standard region (there are nine regions in England, plus Wales). These profiles were constructed from various official data sources. Details of the methodology are given in the Appendix.

Outline of the report

This report includes:

- data on the costs of smoking for three types of GP practice for each of the ten standard regions used in government statistics
- data on the effects of passive smoking on child health and what this means for primary health care teams
- a guide on what the primary care team can do to help smokers stop
- an appendix showing how the data were derived.

1 THE COSTS OF SMOKING TO PRIMARY CARE BY GEOGRAPHICAL REGION

This chapter shows the extent to which smoking affects general practice, giving the costs per general practitioner in the ten major regions of England and Wales. Estimates are given for the annual direct primary care costs of additional GP consultations and prescriptions, and the costs of other NHS treatment, in terms of outpatient visits and inpatient episodes.

Estimates of the additional costs caused by smoking are based on a comparison of the self-reported health service use of current and never smokers from the General Household Survey. For accurate cost calculations, data were combined from the 1988 and 1990 surveys. These cost estimates were applied to predictions of the prevalence of smoking in different regions, and different areas within those regions, based on the 1990 General Household Survey. Figures have been rounded in the tables. More details of the methodology are given in the Appendix.

The total impact of smoking in terms of additional GP consultations, prescriptions, outpatient visits and inpatient episodes has been estimated for England and Wales as a whole. As shown in the table, smoking accounts for an additional 8 million consultations per year and over £140 million direct primary care costs. Including the estimated costs to the NHS, in terms of outpatient and inpatient services that result from these GP consultations, the health service costs of smoking are more than £610 million. These costs only include the effects of smoking on those adults who currently smoke – the costs of smoking in terms of the effects of passive smoking on children are discussed in Chapter 2.

Additional annual costs of smoking in England and Wales

	Number	Costs
Direct primary care costs		
General practice consultations	8 224 000	£ 89 400 000
Prescriptions	7 316 000	£ 52 306 000
Other NHS treatment		
Outpatient visits	4 564 000	£208 880 000
Inpatient episodes	451 000	£260 680 000
Total costs of smoking-related diseases	–	**£611 266 000**

This report illustrates an alternative method for estimating the costs of smoking to that used in previous reports on the costs of smoking.[1, 3] The inpatient costs of smoking in England and Wales estimated in this report

(£261 million) are lower than the total of £325 million estimated previously for England.[1] There are several reasons for the differences in these estimates. Health service use has been derived from the General Household Survey using self reports of individuals living in private households. Figures from the GHS underestimate the total health care use for the population as a whole. Some difference may be due to lower lengths of stay and hence costs for all inpatient care since 1988. Also, the methodology used in this report excludes the health care cost of treating former smokers who have already developed smoking-related illnesses.

A GP with a national average list size of 1911 patients and patients who have smoking rates typical for their age and sex group would incur 297 additional consultations and 265 additional prescriptions each year, as a result of cigarette, cigar and pipe smoking. This additional activity represents a cost of £5125 per year. The resultant use of extra outpatient and inpatient services increases the total health care costs attributable to smoking to over £22 000.

Additional annual costs of smoking for a typical GP (list size 1911, including 1537 adults)

	Number	Costs
Direct primary care costs		
General practice consultations	297	£ 3 233
Prescriptions	265	£ 1 892
Other NHS treatment		
Outpatient visits	165	£ 7 554
Inpatient episodes	16	£ 9 428
Total costs of smoking-related diseases	–	**£22 107**

For each standard region two alternative methods of estimating the proportion of the population currently smoking have been used to produce three different scenarios. Each scenario gives the additional costs of smoking for a GP with an average list size for the region. The first scenario for a 'typical GP' considers the impact for a patient list whose adults have typical rates of smoking for the population of the region.

The second and third scenarios consider alternative types of geographical areas within the region: a rural population and an urban population. Smoking rates in different age, gender and economic groups were calculated from the 1990 General Household Survey. The 1991 Census figures on these characteristics of populations in particular rural and urban areas in each of the standard regions were used to predict the number of current smokers. As may be expected, urban populations tend to have more current smokers and higher cost implications for primary care. However, these are examples based on estimated smoking rates in urban and rural district council areas. Since there will be considerable variation in smoking rates in different areas within these districts, some practices, particularly in inner city areas, will have higher smoking rates and costs.

The following sections contain the following information for each of the ten standard regions of England and Wales:

- current smoking rates based on the 1990 General Household Survey
- direct primary care and other NHS costs per GP with a patient population typical of:
  - the entire region
  - a rural district within the region
  - an urban district within the region.

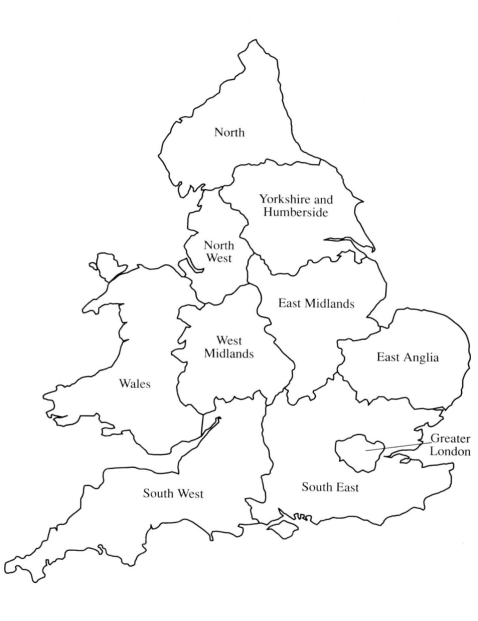

North

Yorkshire and
Humberside

North
West

East Midlands

West
Midlands

East Anglia

Wales

Greater
London

South West

South East

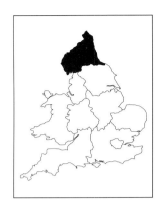

THE NORTH

- 39.4 per cent of men and 30.6 per cent of women smoke cigarettes, pipes or cigars
- among men the highest proportion of smokers, 45.7 per cent, is found in the 35–54 age group
- among women the highest proportion of smokers, 36.6 per cent, is found in the 25–34 age group

Typical GP
(list size 1876, including 1501 adults)

- this practice could expect 264 extra consultations at a cost of £2875 and 275 extra prescriptions at a cost of £1968
- the total annual cost of this is £4843. This does not include the administrative time for the GP to arrange the extra outpatient and inpatient care shown in the table
- the extra consultations alone would take up to 2574 minutes (43 hours)
- the annual cost of additional consultations and prescriptions (direct primary care) to a five-partner practice is £24 215 and in time 215 hours

Additional annual costs of smoking to the practice

	Number	Costs
Direct primary care costs		
General practice consultations	264	£ 2 875
Prescriptions	275	£ 1 968
Other NHS treatment		
Outpatient visits	177	£ 8 088
Inpatient episodes	15	£ 8 893
Total costs of smoking-related diseases	–	**£21 824**

Rural GP
(list size 1876, including 1501 adults)

- this practice could expect 307 extra consultations at a cost of £3332 and 276 extra prescriptions at a cost of £1976
- the total annual cost of this is £5308. This does not include the administrative time for the GP to arrange the extra outpatient and inpatient care shown in the table
- the extra consultations alone would take up to 2994 minutes (50 hours)
- the annual cost of additional consultations and prescriptions (direct primary care) to a five-partner practice is £26 540 and in time 250 hours

Additional annual costs of smoking to the practice

	Number	Costs
Direct primary care costs		
General practice consultations	307	£ 3 332
Prescriptions	276	£ 1 976
Other NHS treatment		
Outpatient visits	159	£ 7 270
Inpatient episodes	16	£ 9 227
Total costs of smoking-related diseases	–	**£21 805**

Urban GP
(list size 1876, including 1501 adults)

- this practice could expect 349 extra consultations at a cost of £3798 and 285 extra prescriptions at a cost of £2034
- the total annual cost of this is £5832. This does not include the administrative time for the GP to arrange the extra outpatient and inpatient care shown in the table
- the extra consultations alone would take up to 3403 minutes (57 hours)
- the annual cost of additional consultations and prescriptions (direct primary care) to a five-partner practice is £29 160 and in time 284 hours

Additional annual costs of smoking to the practice

	Number	Costs
Direct primary care costs		
General practice consultations	349	£ 3 798
Prescriptions	285	£ 2 034
Other NHS treatment		
Outpatient visits	173	£ 7 912
Inpatient episodes	19	£10 799
Total costs of smoking-related diseases	–	**£24 543**

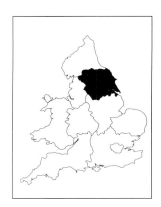

YORKSHIRE AND HUMBERSIDE

- 36.8 per cent of men and 28.0 per cent of women smoke cigarettes, pipes or cigars
- among men the highest proportion of smokers, 44.0 per cent, is found in the 25–34 age group
- among women the highest proportion of smokers, 34.8 per cent, is found in the 35–54 age group

Typical GP
(list size 1878, including 1496 adults)

- this practice could expect 254 extra consultations at a cost of £2765 and 254 extra prescriptions at a cost of £1818
- the total annual cost of this is £4583. This does not include the administrative time for the GP to arrange the extra outpatient and inpatient care shown in the table
- the extra consultations alone would take up to 2479 minutes (41 hours)
- the annual cost of additional consultations and prescriptions (direct primary care) to a five-partner practice is £22 915 and in time 207 hours

Additional annual costs of smoking to the practice

	Number	Costs
Direct primary care costs		
General practice consultations	254	£ 2 765
Prescriptions	254	£ 1 818
Other NHS treatment		
Outpatient visits	146	£ 6 702
Inpatient episodes	14	£ 8 235
Total costs of smoking-related diseases	–	**£19 520**

Rural GP
(list size 1878, including 1496 adults)

- this practice could expect 310 extra consultations at a cost of £3370 and 279 extra prescriptions at a cost of £1998
- the total annual cost of this is £5368. This does not include the administrative time for the GP to arrange the extra outpatient and inpatient care shown in the table
- the extra consultations alone would take up to 2994 minutes (50 hours)
- the annual cost of additional consultations and prescriptions (direct primary care) to a five-partner practice is £26 840 and in time 252 hours

Additional annual costs of smoking to the practice

	Number	Costs
Direct primary care costs		
General practice consultations	310	£ 3 370
Prescriptions	279	£ 1 998
Other NHS treatment		
Outpatient visits	155	£ 7 104
Inpatient episodes	16	£ 9 058
Total costs of smoking-related diseases	–	**£21 530**

Urban GP
(list size 1878, including 1496 adults)

- this practice could expect 352 extra consultations at a cost of £3831 and 287 extra prescriptions at a cost of £2049
- the total annual cost of this is £5880. This does not include the administrative time for the GP to arrange the extra outpatient and inpatient care shown in the table
- the extra consultations alone would take up to 3432 minutes (57 hours)
- the annual cost of additional consultations and prescriptions (direct primary care) to a five-partner practice is £29 400 and in time 286 hours

Additional annual costs of smoking to the practice

	Number	Costs
Direct primary care costs		
General practice consultations	352	£ 3 831
Prescriptions	287	£ 2 049
Other NHS treatment		
Outpatient visits	169	£ 7 737
Inpatient episodes	18	£10 559
Total costs of smoking-related diseases	–	**£24 176**

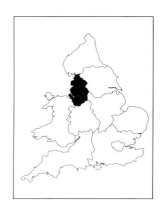

THE NORTH WEST

- 40.4 per cent of men and 32.0 per cent of women smoke cigarettes, pipes or cigars
- among men the highest proportion of smokers, 44.3 per cent, is found in the 16–24 age group
- among women the highest proportion of smokers, 36.8 per cent, is found in the 55–59 age group

Typical GP
(list size 1988, including 1578 adults)

- this practice could expect 369 extra consultations at a cost of £4006 and 315 extra prescriptions at a cost of £2249
- the total annual cost of this is £6255. This does not include the administrative time for the GP to arrange the extra outpatient and inpatient care shown in the table
- the extra consultations alone would take up to 3598 minutes (60 hours)
- the annual cost of additional consultations and prescriptions (direct primary care) to a five-partner practice is £31 275 and in time 300 hours

Additional annual costs of smoking to the practice

	Number	Costs
Direct primary care costs		
General practice consultations	369	£ 4 006
Prescriptions	315	£ 2 249
Other NHS treatment		
Outpatient visits	190	£ 8 716
Inpatient episodes	19	£10 875
Total costs of smoking-related diseases	–	**£25 846**

Rural GP
(list size 1988, including 1578 adults)

- this practice could expect 357 extra consultations at a cost of £3881 and 308 extra prescriptions at a cost of £2203
- the total annual cost of this is £6084. This does not include the administrative time for the GP to arrange the extra outpatient and inpatient care shown in the table
- the extra consultations alone would take up to 3481 minutes (58 hours)
- the annual cost of additional consultations and prescriptions (direct primary care) to a five-partner practice is £30 420 and in time 290 hours

Additional annual costs of smoking to the practice

	Number	Costs
Direct primary care costs		
General practice consultations	357	£ 3 881
Prescriptions	308	£ 2 203
Other NHS treatment		
Outpatient visits	175	£ 7 992
Inpatient episodes	18	£10 491
Total costs of smoking-related diseases	–	**£24 567**

Urban GP
(list size 1988, including 1578 adults)

- this practice could expect 408 extra consultations at a cost of £4431 and 309 extra prescriptions at a cost of £2208
- the total annual cost of this is £6639. This does not include the administrative time for the GP to arrange the extra outpatient and inpatient care shown in the table
- the extra consultations alone would take up to 3979 minutes (66 hours)
- the annual cost of additional consultations and prescriptions (direct primary care) to a five-partner practice is £33 195 and in time 332 hours

Additional annual costs of smoking to the practice

	Number	Costs
Direct primary care costs		
General practice consultations	408	£ 4 431
Prescriptions	309	£ 2 208
Other NHS treatment		
Outpatient visits	196	£ 8 957
Inpatient episodes	22	£12 746
Total costs of smoking-related diseases	–	**£28 342**

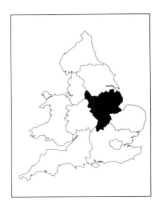

EAST MIDLANDS

- 35.0 per cent of men and 26.7 per cent of women smoke cigarettes, pipes or cigars
- among men the highest proportion of smokers, 42.5 per cent, is found in the 25–34 age group
- among women the highest proportion of smokers, 33.3 per cent, is found in the 16–24 age group

Typical GP
(list size 1930, including 1551 adults)

- this practice could expect 283 extra consultations at a cost of £3074 and 234 extra prescriptions at a cost of £1676
- the total annual cost of this is £4750. This does not include the administrative time for the GP to arrange the extra outpatient and inpatient care shown in the table
- the extra consultations alone would take up to 2760 minutes (46 hours)
- the annual cost of additional consultations and prescriptions (direct primary care) to a five-partner practice is £23 750 and in time 230 hours

Additional annual costs of smoking to the practice

	Number	Costs
Direct primary care costs		
General practice consultations	283	£ 3 074
Prescriptions	234	£ 1 676
Other NHS treatment		
Outpatient visits	160	£ 7 345
Inpatient episodes	17	£ 9 724
Total costs of smoking-related diseases	–	**£21 819**

Rural GP
(list size 1930, including 1551 adults)

- this practice could expect 349 extra consultations at a cost of £3799 and 302 extra prescriptions at a cost of £2156
- the total annual cost of this is £5955. This does not include the administrative time for the GP to arrange the extra outpatient and inpatient care shown in the table
- the extra consultations alone would take up to 3403 minutes (57 hours)
- the annual cost of additional consultations and prescriptions (direct primary care) to a five-partner practice is £29 775 and in time 284 hours

Additional annual costs of smoking to the practice

	Number	Costs
Direct primary care costs		
General practice consultations	349	£ 3 799
Prescriptions	302	£ 2 156
Other NHS treatment		
Outpatient visits	165	£ 7 535
Inpatient episodes	17	£ 9 841
Total costs of smoking-related diseases	–	**£23 331**

Urban GP
(list size 1930, including 1551 adults)

- this practice could expect 388 extra consultations at a cost of £4221 and 298 extra prescriptions at a cost of £2128
- the total annual cost of this is £6349. This does not include the administrative time for the GP to arrange the extra outpatient and inpatient care shown in the table
- the extra consultations alone would take up to 3784 minutes (63 hours)
- the annual cost of additional consultations and prescriptions (direct primary care) to a five-partner practice is £31 745 and in time 315 hours

Additional annual costs of smoking to the practice

	Number	Costs
Direct primary care costs		
General practice consultations	388	£ 4 221
Prescriptions	298	£ 2 128
Other NHS treatment		
Outpatient visits	187	£ 8 571
Inpatient episodes	21	£12 060
Total costs of smoking-related diseases	–	**£26 980**

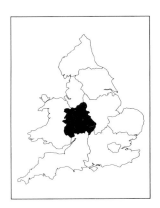

WEST MIDLANDS

- 38.0 per cent of men and 27.7 per cent of women smoke cigarettes, pipes or cigars
- among men the highest proportion of smokers, 41.8 per cent, is found in the 25–34 age group
- among women the highest proportion of smokers, 39.1 per cent, is found in the 16–24 age group

Typical GP
(list size 1969, including 1567 adults)

- this practice could expect 324 extra consultations at a cost of £3524 and 273 extra prescriptions at a cost of £1950
- the total annual cost of this is £5474. This does not include the administrative time for the GP to arrange the extra outpatient and inpatient care shown in the table
- the extra consultations alone would take up to 3159 minutes (53 hours)
- the annual cost of additional consultations and prescriptions (direct primary care) to a five-partner practice is £27 370 and in time 263 hours

Additional annual costs of smoking to the practice

	Number	Costs
Direct primary care costs		
General practice consultations	324	£ 3 524
Prescriptions	273	£ 1 950
Other NHS treatment		
Outpatient visits	175	£ 8 023
Inpatient episodes	18	£10 340
Total costs of smoking-related diseases	–	**£23 837**

Rural GP
(list size 1969, including 1567 adults)

- this practice could expect 325 extra consultations at a cost of £3534 and 294 extra prescriptions at a cost of £2104
- the total annual cost of this is £5638. This does not include the administrative time for the GP to arrange the extra outpatient and inpatient care shown in the table
- the extra consultations alone would take up to 3169 minutes (53 hours)
- the annual cost of additional consultations and prescriptions (direct primary care) to a five-partner practice is £28 190 and in time 264 hours

Additional annual costs of smoking to the practice

	Number	Costs
Direct primary care costs		
General practice consultations	325	£ 3 534
Prescriptions	294	£ 2 104
Other NHS treatment		
Outpatient visits	163	£ 7 452
Inpatient episodes	16	£ 9 269
Total costs of smoking-related diseases	–	**£22 359**

Urban GP
(list size 1969, including 1567 adults)

- this practice could expect 391 extra consultations at a cost of £4245 and 306 extra prescriptions at a cost of £2188
- the total annual cost of this is £6433. This does not include the administrative time for the GP to arrange the extra outpatient and inpatient care shown in the table
- the extra consultations alone would take up to 3813 minutes (64 hours)
- the annual cost of additional consultations and prescriptions (direct primary care) to a five-partner practice is £32 165 and in time 318 hours

Additional annual costs of smoking to the practice

	Number	Costs
Direct primary care costs		
General practice consultations	391	£ 4 245
Prescriptions	306	£ 2 188
Other NHS treatment		
Outpatient visits	187	£ 8 543
Inpatient episodes	21	£11 948
Total costs of smoking-related diseases	–	**£26 924**

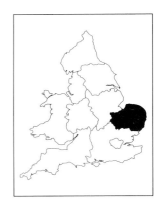

EAST ANGLIA

- 34.3 per cent of men and 23.2 per cent of women smoke cigarettes, pipes or cigars
- among men the highest proportion of smokers, 41.3 per cent, is found in the 65–74 age group
- among women the highest proportion of smokers, 41.4 per cent, is found in the 16–24 age group

Typical GP
(list size 1793, including 1448 adults)

- this practice could expect 286 extra consultations at a cost of £3106 and 230 extra prescriptions at a cost of £1641
- the total annual cost of this is £4747. This does not include the administrative time for the GP to arrange the extra outpatient and inpatient care shown in the table
- the extra consultations alone would take up to 2789 minutes (46 hours)
- the annual cost of additional consultations and prescriptions (direct primary care) to a five-partner practice is £23 735 and in time 232 hours

Additional annual costs of smoking to the practice

	Number	Costs
Direct primary care costs		
General practice consultations	286	£ 3 106
Prescriptions	230	£ 1 641
Other NHS treatment		
Outpatient visits	175	£ 8 008
Inpatient episodes	18	£10 145
Total costs of smoking-related diseases	–	**£22 900**

Rural GP
(list size 1793, including 1448 adults)

- this practice could expect 331 extra consultations at a cost of £3595 and 263 extra prescriptions at a cost of £1881
- the total annual cost of this is £5476. This does not include the administrative time for the GP to arrange the extra outpatient and inpatient care shown in the table
- the extra consultations alone would take up to 3228 minutes (54 hours)
- the annual cost of additional consultations and prescriptions (direct primary care) to a five-partner practice is £27 380 and in time 269 hours

Additional annual costs of smoking to the practice

	Number	Costs
Direct primary care costs		
General practice consultations	331	£ 3 595
Prescriptions	263	£ 1 881
Other NHS treatment		
Outpatient visits	161	£ 7 351
Inpatient episodes	18	£10 140
Total costs of smoking-related diseases	–	**£22 967**

Urban GP
(list size 1793, including 1448 adults)

- this practice could expect 341 extra consultations at a cost of £3703 and 268 extra prescriptions at a cost of £1913
- the total annual cost of this is £5616. This does not include the administrative time for the GP to arrange the extra outpatient and inpatient care shown in the table
- the extra consultations alone would take up to 3325 minutes (55 hours)
- the annual cost of additional consultations and prescriptions (direct primary care) to a five-partner practice is £28 080 and in time 277 hours

Additional annual costs of smoking to the practice

	Number	Costs
Direct primary care costs		
General practice consultations	341	£ 3 703
Prescriptions	268	£ 1 913
Other NHS treatment		
Outpatient visits	166	£ 7 615
Inpatient episodes	18	£10 424
Total costs of smoking-related diseases	–	**£23 655**

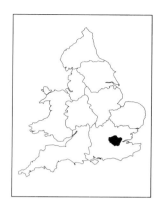

GREATER LONDON

- 37.5 per cent of men and 28.2 per cent of women smoke cigarettes, pipes or cigars
- among men the highest proportion of smokers, 42.9 per cent, is found in the 35–54 age group
- among women the highest proportion of smokers, 36.0 per cent, is found in the 25–34 age group

Typical GP
(list size 2035, including 1654 adults)

- this practice could expect 317 extra consultations at a cost of £3443 and 275 extra prescriptions at a cost of £1963
- the total annual cost of this is £5406. This does not include the administrative time for the GP to arrange the extra outpatient and inpatient care shown in the table
- the extra consultations alone would take up to 3091 minutes (52 hours)
- the annual cost of additional consultations and prescriptions (direct primary care) to a five-partner practice is £27 030 and in time 258 hours

Additional annual costs of smoking to the practice

	Number	Costs
Direct primary care costs		
General practice consultations	317	£ 3 443
Prescriptions	275	£ 1 963
Other NHS treatment		
Outpatient visits	176	£ 8 052
Inpatient episodes	19	£10 844
Total costs of smoking-related diseases	–	**£24 302**

Rural GP
(list size 2035, including 1654 adults)

- this practice could expect 365 extra consultations at a cost of £3967 and 311 extra prescriptions at a cost of £2223
- the total annual cost of this is £6190. This does not include the administrative time for the GP to arrange the extra outpatient and inpatient care shown in the table
- the extra consultations alone would take up to 3559 minutes (59 hours)
- the annual cost of additional consultations and prescriptions (direct primary care) to a five-partner practice is £30 950 and in time 297 hours

Additional annual costs of smoking to the practice

	Number	Costs
Direct primary care costs		
General practice consultations	365	£ 3 967
Prescriptions	311	£ 2 223
Other NHS treatment		
Outpatient visits	177	£ 8 116
Inpatient episodes	19	£10 753
Total costs of smoking-related diseases	–	**£25 059**

Urban GP
(list size 2035, including 1654 adults)

- this practice could expect 411 extra consultations at a cost of £4469 and 303 extra prescriptions at a cost of £2165
- the total annual cost of this is £6634. This does not include the administrative time for the GP to arrange the extra outpatient and inpatient care shown in the table
- the extra consultations alone would take up to 4007 minutes (67 hours)
- the annual cost of additional consultations and prescriptions (direct primary care) to a five-partner practice is £33 170 and in time 334 hours

Additional annual costs of smoking to the practice

	Number	Costs
Direct primary care costs		
General practice consultations	411	£ 4 469
Prescriptions	303	£ 2 165
Other NHS treatment		
Outpatient visits	200	£ 9 153
Inpatient episodes	24	£13 674
Total costs of smoking-related diseases	–	**£29 461**

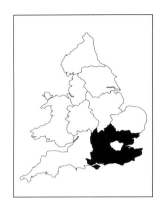

THE SOUTH EAST

- 36.9 per cent of men and 26.2 per cent of women smoke cigarettes, pipes or cigars
- among men the highest proportion of smokers, 41.6 per cent, is found in the 25–34 age group
- among women the highest proportion of smokers, 41.6 per cent, is found in the 16–24 age group

Typical GP
(list size 1965, including 1604 adults)

- this practice could expect 316 extra consultations at a cost of £3431 and 272 extra prescriptions at a cost of £1942
- the total annual cost of this is £5373. This does not include the administrative time for the GP to arrange the extra outpatient and inpatient care shown in the table
- the extra consultations alone would take up to 3081 minutes (51 hours)
- the annual cost of additional consultations and prescriptions (direct primary care) to a five-partner practice is £26 865 and in time 257 hours

Additional annual costs of smoking to the practice

	Number	Costs
Direct primary care costs		
General practice consultations	316	£ 3 431
Prescriptions	272	£ 1 942
Other NHS treatment		
Outpatient visits	172	£ 7 866
Inpatient episodes	16	£ 9 419
Total costs of smoking-related diseases	–	**£22 658**

Rural GP
(list size 1965, including 1604 adults)

- this practice could expect 351 extra consultations at a cost of £3819 and 305 extra prescriptions at a cost of £2180
- the total annual cost of this is £5999. This does not include the administrative time for the GP to arrange the extra outpatient and inpatient care shown in the table
- the extra consultations alone would take up to 3423 minutes (57 hours)
- the annual cost of additional consultations and prescriptions (direct primary care) to a five-partner practice is £29 995 and in time 285 hours

Additional annual costs of smoking to the practice

	Number	Costs
Direct primary care costs		
General practice consultations	351	£ 3 819
Prescriptions	305	£ 2 180
Other NHS treatment		
Outpatient visits	172	£ 7 883
Inpatient episodes	18	£10 267
Total costs of smoking-related diseases	–	**£24 149**

Urban GP
(list size 1965, including 1604 adults)

- this practice could expect 351 extra consultations at a cost of £3813 and 287 extra prescriptions at a cost of £2054
- the total annual cost of this is £5867. This does not include the administrative time for the GP to arrange the extra outpatient and inpatient care shown in the table
- the extra consultations alone would take up to 3423 minutes (57 hours)
- the annual cost of additional consultations and prescriptions (direct primary care) to a five-partner practice is £29 335 and in time 285 hours

Additional annual costs of smoking to the practice

	Number	Costs
Direct primary care costs		
General practice consultations	351	£ 3 813
Prescriptions	287	£ 2 054
Other NHS treatment		
Outpatient visits	176	£ 8 075
Inpatient episodes	19	£10 864
Total costs of smoking-related diseases	–	**£24 806**

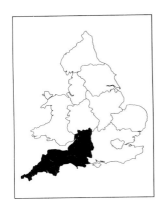

THE SOUTH WEST

- 36.2 per cent of men and 24.0 per cent of women smoke cigarettes, pipes or cigars
- among men the highest proportion of smokers, 44.9 per cent, is found in the 35–54 age group
- among women the highest proportion of smokers, 37.0 per cent, is found in the 16–24 age group

Typical GP
(list size 1741, including 1413 adults)

- this practice could expect 244 extra consultations at a cost of £2654 and 230 extra prescriptions at a cost of £1647
- the total annual cost of this is £4301. This does not include the administrative time for the GP to arrange the extra outpatient and inpatient care shown in the table
- the extra consultations alone would take up to 2379 minutes (40 hours)
- the annual cost of additional consultations and prescriptions (direct primary care) to a five-partner practice is £21 505 and in time 198 hours

Additional annual costs of smoking to the practice

	Number	Costs
Direct primary care costs		
General practice consultations	244	£ 2 654
Prescriptions	230	£ 1 647
Other NHS treatment		
Outpatient visits	141	£ 6 453
Inpatient episodes	14	£ 7 958
Total costs of smoking-related diseases	–	**£18 712**

Rural GP
(list size 1741, including 1413 adults)

- this practice could expect 300 extra consultations at a cost of £3266 and 261 extra prescriptions at a cost of £1863
- the total annual cost of this is £5129. This does not include the administrative time for the GP to arrange the extra outpatient and inpatient care shown in the table
- the extra consultations alone would take up to 2925 minutes (49 hours)
- the annual cost of additional consultations and prescriptions (direct primary care) to a five-partner practice is £25 645 and in time 262 hours

Additional annual costs of smoking to the practice

	Number	Costs
Direct primary care costs		
General practice consultations	300	£ 3 266
Prescriptions	261	£ 1 863
Other NHS treatment		
Outpatient visits	151	£ 6 927
Inpatient episodes	15	£ 8 883
Total costs of smoking-related diseases	–	**£20 939**

Urban GP
(list size 1741, including 1413 adults)

- this practice could expect 325 extra consultations at a cost of £3530 and 261 extra prescriptions at a cost of £1866
- the total annual cost of this is £5396. This does not include the administrative time for the GP to arrange the extra outpatient and inpatient care shown in the table
- the extra consultations alone would take up to 3169 minutes (53 hours)
- the annual cost of additional consultations and prescriptions (direct primary care) to a five-partner practice is £26 980 and in time 264 hours

Additional annual costs of smoking to the practice

	Number	Costs
Direct primary care costs		
General practice consultations	325	£ 3 530
Prescriptions	261	£ 1 866
Other NHS treatment		
Outpatient visits	160	£ 7 331
Inpatient episodes	17	£10 024
Total costs of smoking-related diseases	–	**£22 751**

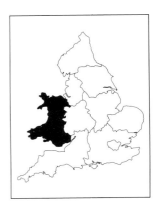

WALES

- 35.8 per cent of men and 30.2 per cent of women smoke cigarettes, pipes or cigars
- among men the highest proportion of smokers, 45.7 per cent, is found in the 35–54 age group
- among women the highest proportion of smokers, 41.2 per cent, is found in the 55–59 age group

Typical GP
(list size 1743, including 1395 adults)

- this practice could expect 267 extra consultations at a cost of £2903 and 259 extra prescriptions at a cost of £1854
- the total annual cost of this is £4757. This does not include the administrative time for the GP to arrange the extra outpatient and inpatient care shown in the table
- the extra consultations alone would take up to 2604 minutes (43 hours)
- the annual cost of additional consultations and prescriptions (direct primary care) to a five-partner practice is £23 785 and in time 217 hours

Additional annual costs of smoking to the practice

	Number	Costs
Direct primary care costs		
General practice consultations	267	£ 2 903
Prescriptions	259	£ 1 854
Other NHS treatment		
Outpatient visits	124	£ 5 690
Inpatient episodes	14	£ 7 888
Total costs of smoking-related diseases	–	**£18 335**

Rural GP
(list size 1395, based on 5 GPs)

- this practice could expect 307 extra consultations at a cost of £3341 and 265 extra prescriptions at a cost of £1894
- the total annual cost of this is £5235. This does not include the administrative time for the GP to arrange the extra outpatient and inpatient care shown in the table
- the extra consultations alone would take up to 2994 minutes (50 hours)
- the annual cost of additional consultations and prescriptions (direct primary care) to a five-partner practice is £26 175 and in time 250 hours

Additional annual costs of smoking to the practice

	Number	Costs
Direct primary care costs		
General practice consultations	307	£ 3 341
Prescriptions	265	£ 1 894
Other NHS treatment		
Outpatient visits	154	£ 7 056
Inpatient episodes	16	£ 9 144
Total costs of smoking-related diseases	–	**£21 435**

Urban GP
(list size 1743, including 1395 adults)

- this practice could expect 329 extra consultations at a cost of £3576 and 267 extra prescriptions at a cost of £1911
- the total annual cost of this is £5487. This does not include the administrative time for the GP to arrange the extra outpatient and inpatient care shown in the table
- the extra consultations alone would take up to 3208 minutes (53 hours)
- the annual cost of additional consultations and prescriptions (direct primary care) to a five-partner practice is £27 435 and in time 267 hours

Additional annual costs of smoking to the practice

	Number	Costs
Direct primary care costs		
General practice consultations	329	£ 3 576
Prescriptions	267	£ 1 911
Other NHS treatment		
Outpatient visits	160	£ 7 323
Inpatient episodes	17	£ 9 983
Total costs of smoking-related diseases	–	**£22 793**

2 PASSIVE SMOKING AND CHILDREN

Smoking does not only damage the health of those who smoke. The effects on the unborn child from maternal smoking have been well documented, and can provide a powerful motivation to some prospective parents to stop: *I first gave up when I was expecting my daughter. When I first found out I was pregnant I cut down to about four or five a day, then within a couple of months I just stopped completely. That was it, my baby was more important because I had a great deal of trouble getting pregnant anyway. She was more important than anything else in the world. I just didn't start again.* More recent reports have highlighted the effects on infants and children.[3] Passive smoking causes acute irritation of the eyes, throat and respiratory tract. The evidence strongly suggests that passive smoking is responsible for chronic middle-ear disease and for the aggravation of asthma. There is evidence, though not yet conclusive, of a link between parental smoking and childhood respiratory illness.

As highlighted in *The Smoking Epidemic: a Manifesto for Action*[3] a large number of children are exposed to smoke through their parents' smoking, something the children themselves are becoming more sensitive to: *It got to the stage when she was having her breakfast and things upstairs so she didn't have to stay with us while we smoked. A little extreme perhaps, but quite a sobering experience.* In this report we examine the potential link between having smokers in the household and the children's use of health services.

Using data from the 1990 General Household Survey, it can be seen that 51 per cent of children live in a household with a person who smokes. Across the country children in the South East are the least likely to live in a household with a smoker (46 per cent) whereas in Wales over 57 per cent of children live with an adult smoker.

Costs of the effects of passive smoking on children

Children in households with a smoker visit the GP more often, have more prescriptions, more outpatient visits and more inpatient stays than children in non-smoking households. Using prevalence estimates from the 1990 General Household Survey, and estimates of health service use from the 1988 and 1990 General Household Surveys combined, the annual costs to the NHS were calculated at over £140 million. These costs were based on the difference between use of health services by children exposed to passive smoking in the household and by those who are not. Figures are calculated for England and Wales and for children 0 to 15 (see Appendix for the details of the methodology). Figures have been rounded in the tables.

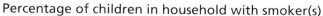

Percentage of children in household with smoker(s)

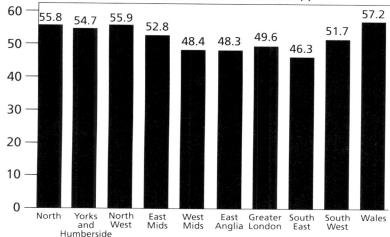

Passive smoking in England and Wales

Region

Annual costs of the additional health care for children who live with smokers in England and Wales

	Number	Costs
Direct primary care costs		
General practice consultations	1 533 000	£ 16 668 000
Prescriptions	2 013 000	£ 14 390 000
Other NHS treatment		
Outpatient visits	468 000	£ 21 403 000
Inpatient episodes	157 000	£ 90 959 000
Total additional costs	–	**£143 421 000**

Taking a GP with a typical list size of 1911, containing approximately 374 children, it is estimated that there would be a total of 55 extra consultations per year for the children in households with a smoker. These consultations would take up to 536 minutes or 9 hours. The resource costs to the GP of the extra consultations and prescriptions would be £1124 and the other NHS treatment £4065 each year.

Annual costs of the additional health care for children who live with smokers for a typical GP

	Number	Costs
Direct primary care costs		
General practice consultations	55	£ 603
Prescriptions	73	£ 521
Other NHS treatment		
Outpatient visits	17	£ 774
Inpatient episodes	6	£3 291
Total additional costs	–	**£5 189**

In summary, passive smoking is a serious health issue for children, with large potential costs to the NHS. These are additional to the direct costs of smoking incurred by adult smokers detailed in the first two editions of *The Smoking Epidemic*[1,3] and in Chapter 1 of this report. Furthermore, it may be worth remembering that we have not considered the costs of passive smoking to adults or to the unborn child.

Clearly then, helping smokers to stop needs to be a top priority for the health care system, especially in primary care. Chapter 3 contains some simple guidelines for the practice team.

3 HELPING SMOKERS STOP: GUIDE-LINES FOR THE PRACTICE TEAM

The central role of the practice team

Simple advice and support from the practice team is potentially one of the most effective strategies for reducing smoking prevalence. A protocol appears below which all practices could adopt to achieve this. The data in this report indicate the huge benefit such a strategy would produce in primary care in the long term.

Our message to the practice team is that if they help smokers to stop they will:

- improve the quality of the smokers' lives
- eventually free time which can be devoted to other activities.

Ex-smokers really experience benefits from stopping. Here's what some ex-smokers said: *Being able to breathe better was one of the first signs – not getting breathless. I can walk further and I ride a bike now. Rather than sitting in the house gasping for a cigarette, I get out and about. In the five months since we gave up smoking we've managed to get satellite television and a camcorder all for cash and that is simply for cigarettes, put into a jar.*

The practice team is in a unique position:

- smokers come to them (across the UK about 250 000 smokers see their GP every day)
- research shows that smokers expect advice on smoking and suggests that silence on the topic is interpreted as condoning it [5]
- the evidence shows that advice from primary care professionals *is* effective in helping smokers stop [6]
- more training is becoming available for the primary care team to improve cessation counselling skills.

During a conversation about the benefits of giving up smoking a GP was frustrated to hear the smoker say: *My angina has got nothing to do with smoking, or the cardiologist would have told me to stop.* Conversely firm, clear advice from a health professional linking the smoker's condition to their smoking can have a powerful effect: *I was very overweight and I had high blood pressure, and it really was the doctor's warning that I was heading for a heart attack and all the rest of it! My heart kept beating different beats. I ended up having sleepless nights and panicking. I thought 'No this is stupid' so I decided to give up.*

Evidence that general practice intervention is effective

Russell and his colleagues showed in 1979 that simple advice plus a leaflet and the promise of follow-up persuaded 5 per cent of smokers to stop at one year follow-up. The figure in the non-intervention control group was 0.3 per cent.[7] Although 5 per cent might seem a poor result, in fact it is excellent. It would mean about 100 ex-smokers in a year in a five-partner practice, hundreds of thousands nationwide – an *enormously* worthwhile result. Further research has confirmed these results and shown that with the addition of nicotine replacement therapy, success rates are roughly doubled, to around 10 per cent.[8] Success rates of nicotine gum and patch are similar so that the choice between them depends on practical considerations like the ability to chew and ease of use.

Most smokers try to stop several times before eventually succeeding and research has shown that they go through a number of stages during this process. The first stage is thinking about stopping, from which they move on to preparing to stop, trying to stop, stopping, possibly relapsing, and eventually maintaining abstinence. This model has been called the 'Stages of change' model and was developed by two psychologists, Prochaska and DiClemente.[9] The Health Education Authority's training course for practice nurses (and other PHC professionals) Helping People Change is based on the model.[10] According to the model a brief intervention which *appeared* to fail may have succeeded, by helping the smoker move from one stage to the next, as this smoker's story illustrates: *I've given up smoking hundreds of times before. It's really quite easy! It's the staying stopped that's not. It's different this time.*

The process of change

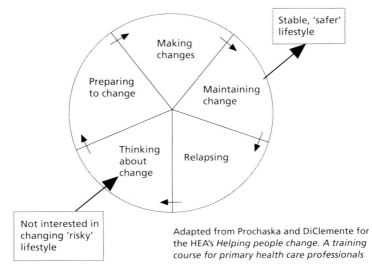

Making changes

Stable, 'safer' lifestyle

Preparing to change

Maintaining change

Thinking about change

Relapsing

Not interested in changing 'risky' lifestyle

Adapted from Prochaska and DiClemente for the HEA's *Helping people change. A training course for primary health care professionals*

The message is that if the first intervention appears to have no effect it is worth trying again. This approach has many benefits. It is client centred and means that in effect the health professional cannot 'fail'. Their responsibility is to find out what stage the smoker is at and then give the appropriate intervention. The model means that smokers cannot be forced to stop if they are not ready, so that the health professional need not feel obliged to attempt to force this change. Acknowledging that someone is not ready to change and perhaps giving a leaflet might sow the seeds for eventual change, a change the practice team is in a unique position to assist. This approach also improves the confidence of the health professional. Because it emphasises giving an intervention appropriate to the stage the smoker is at it is likely to be well received.

This quote shows how supportive the practice team can be: *We went straight to the practice nurse, but saw the GP in passing. The nurse did the physical and the nurse did all the counselling. The patches were a tremendous help. We had both given up smoking before, separately. I think if we'd both given up smoking together without using the patches, we'd have been divorced by now.*

Health promotion in general practice

The protocol shown in the flow chart on pp.34–35 could be adopted by practices wishing to be more active in smoking cessation. All three bands of the 1993 health promotion contract specify that practices also focus on priority groups, try to reach non-attenders, and collaborate with other agencies. Since smoking-related damage is proportional to total smoke exposure, the highest risk group are heavier smokers who have smoked for a long time, i.e. are older. Older smokers are likely to be more motivated to stop (cessation rates rise with age, especially over 30) and so should probably be the main priority group for intervention. They are likely to include some smokers in the priority groups suggested in the new contract: pregnant women, women on oral contraceptives, smokers with children, those with hypertension, respiratory or cardiovascular disease, and those about to undergo surgery.

What you can do

On the following two pages simple guidelines for the practice team are offered in the form of a suggested protocol to be adopted during consultations, plus additional activities within the primary care team as a whole.

Guidelines for the practice team

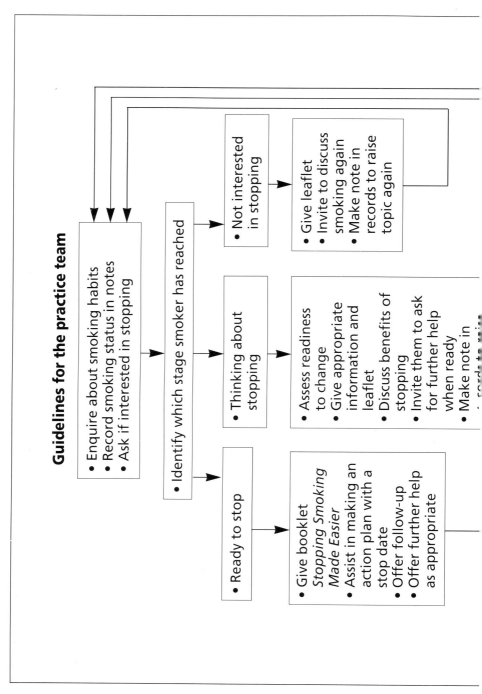

- Enquire about smoking habits
- Record smoking status in notes
- Ask if interested in stopping

- Identify which stage smoker has reached

Not interested in stopping
- Give leaflet
- Invite to discuss smoking again
- Make note in records to raise topic again

Thinking about stopping
- Assess readiness to change
- Give appropriate information and leaflet
- Discuss benefits of stopping
- Invite them to ask for further help when ready
- Make note in records to raise

Ready to stop
- Give booklet *Stopping Smoking Made Easier*
- Assist in making an action plan with a stop date
- Offer follow-up
- Offer further help as appropriate

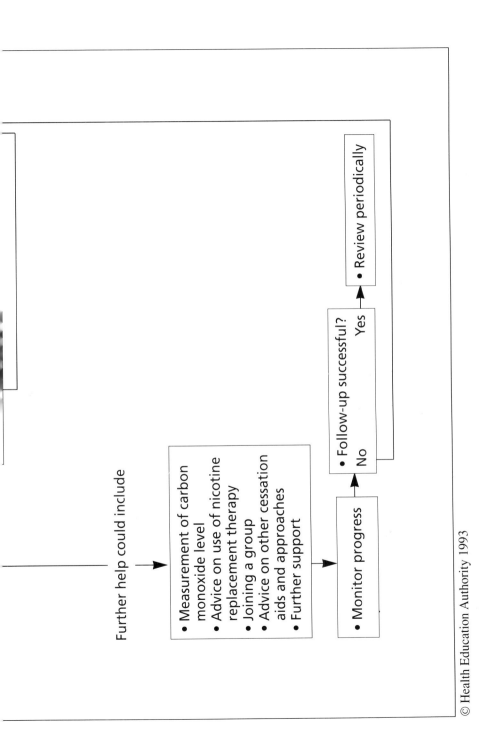

Further help could include

- Measurement of carbon monoxide level
- Advice on use of nicotine replacement therapy
- Joining a group
- Advice on other cessation aids and approaches
- Further support

↓

- Monitor progress

→

- Follow-up successful?

No   Yes

- Review periodically

Within the primary care team

- Make sure your practice has sufficient supplies of appropriate literature.
- Establish a smoke-free policy in the practice.
- Agree a clear 'message' to be adopted when dealing with all initial enquiries and involve the reception staff in what you are trying to achieve.
- Establish clear roles. For example the GP could raise the issue and then refer to the practice nurse for further advice and support. Practice manager could order leaflets.
- Review the staff training needs implied by all this and seek appropiate training.
- Establish links with other agencies able to support this strategy (for example, health promotion departments). You may wish to link up with other local surgeries to hold cessation groups in rotation.

Training and resources

Training

Various individuals and agencies will be able to offer advice and help on smoking cessation and training. These may include: local health promotion units, FHSA primary care facilitators, practice nurse advisers, individual consultants, national organisations like ASH, Quit, Royal College of Nursing, Royal College of General Practitioners, and national health promotion agencies like the Health Education Authority and Health Promotion Authority for Wales. Of particular relevance is the HEA training course for practice nurses and other members of the primary health care team, Helping People Change, details of which can be obtained from the HEA Primary Health Care Unit in Oxford (0865 226061).

Resources

The Health Education Authority and other health promotion agencies also publish leaflets and booklets for smokers designed to support the stepwise approach outlined in the flowchart on pages 34-5.

The HEA's information centre has a comprehensive list of smoking resources. Details from: Health Promotion Information Centre, Hamilton House, Mabledon Place, London WC1H 9TX (071-383 3833).

The HEA's HELIOS project aims to support local health promotion units in their work against smoking, and links the work of national agencies with local workers. It also produces an agencies and resources guide. Details from: HEA HELIOS Project, University of the West of England, Bristol BS6 6UZ (0272 238317).

Useful publications for the primary care team:

Help your patient stop (booklet, BMA)
Thinking about stopping? (leaflet, HEA)
Stopping smoking made easier (leaflet, HEA)
Stopping smoking and carbon monoxide (leaflet, Bedfont Scientific Ltd)
Do you want to stop? (poster, Bedfont Scientific Ltd)
Smoking: the facts (booklet, HEA)
Better living, better life (folder, Knowledge House).

APPENDIX

Overview

The methodology adopted in the first two editions of *The Smoking Epidemic*[1,3] was based on the proportion of each disease, for example lung cancer, attributable to smoking. For inpatient stays, data are collected on the diagnosed disease. However, recent information is not available for other health service use such as outpatient attendances or consultations with general practitioners. An alternative methodology is to compare the use of different services by smokers and non-smokers and this was the methodology used in this study.

The advantage of using differences by smoking status is that the figures are based on behaviour rather than proportions drawn from epidemiological and clinical studies. The disadvantage in comparing smokers and non-smokers is that some of the differences may be due to other characteristics of the two groups, for example, in drinking behaviour or housing conditions. Some studies[11,12] have attempted to adjust data for different characteristics but in one study[12] the effects were found to be small. In this study adjustments were made for age and sex so that potential excess costs were not exaggerated, but no attempt was made to adjust for other factors.

Prevalence figures are primarily based on the 1990 General Household Survey (GHS). To avoid problems with small sample sizes, data from both the 1988 and 1990 GHS were combined for the estimation of health service use by smokers and non-smokers in different age and sex groups, and in the estimation of regional variations in the exposure of children to passive smoking in the household (Chapter 2). The estimates are prevalence rather than incidence based, i.e. the extra costs refer to the situation that *occurred* in that year rather than those that would be *predicted* from forecasting the impact over future years from a change in smoking rates.

The use and cost of health services

The GHS contains questions for each adult about their use of health services in four areas: the number of visits to a doctor in the last two weeks; whether a prescription was received at each doctor consultation; the visits made as an outpatient to a hospital in the last 3 months; and the number of inpatient episodes in the last year. Similar questions are asked about the use of these services by children (those younger than 16 years old) in the household. These figures were converted to an annual amount.

In converting numbers and events to costs, average figures for the length of the visit to the general practitioner, the cost of the prescription and the length of stay in a hospital were used. The average length of a consultation with a GP was estimated to be 9.8 minutes, based on a weighted average of the length of surgery and home visits in the DHSS/General Medical Services survey of 1987. To convert numbers to costs the following figures and sources were used:

Cost of a GP visit[13] (1993/94)	£ 10.87
Cost of a prescription[14] (1991/92)	£ 7.15
Outpatient attendance[15] (1990/91)	£ 45.77
Inpatient episodes[15] (1990/91)	£577.70

As indicated, the figures are taken from a variety of sources and relate to different time periods but can be taken as the minimum costs for 1993/94.

Smoking status

(a) Adult smoking

Three main groups were defined: current smokers, never smokers and former smokers. In this study a broader definition of smoking status was taken than in previous reports. Smokers include all those who smoke cigarettes, pipes or cigars. Jarvis and Jackson[16] suggest that some giving up cigarettes may switch to pipes or cigars with additional health risk to those who had only ever smoked (and not inhaled) pipes or cigars. This group may affect comparisons. Also children may be affected whatever is smoked.

(b) Children and passive smoking

The calculations for children exposed to passive smoking included all adults in the households whether or not they were the child's parents. Children throughout the report are defined as those aged 15 or younger.

Smoking status and additional health service use and costs

(a) Costs of passive smoking among children

To calculate the figures presented in Chapter 2 the health service use of children in households with a current smoker was compared to the use of health services by children in households with no current adult smoker. Some of the 'non-smoking' households may contain recent quitters and their children may still suffer some smoking-related effects. Similarly, some current smokers may only smoke at work or in the evenings and, therefore, never or very rarely in front of the children. Although these possibilities may bias the estimates downwards the effects are likely to be small. Alternatively, the costs of passive smoking may be exaggerated because of other differences between the households, particularly income, which may affect the child's health.

(b) Costs of smoking among adults

Many studies have combined current smokers with former smokers to esti-
mate the costs of smoking-related diseases.[11] This allows for the effect of
chronic smoking-related diseases which may necessitate quitting smoking
for some individuals. However, the comparison between ever smokers and
never smokers may exaggerate the costs attributable to smoking behaviour.
In this study the basic tables are based on the difference between current
and never smokers. Rather than using an average figure the basic calculations were broken down by gender and age groups.

For men of all ages, current smokers had more visits to their GPs, had
more prescriptions, outpatient, inpatient visits than never smokers. For
women the figures were more complex. For the 25- to 34-year-old group
women never smokers had slightly more GP visits and received more prescriptions than current smokers. This may, however, reflect different preg-
nancy rates between the two groups. Among older women there were also
some 'perverse' results with current smokers using less of a health care
item than never smokers. There were, however, only small numbers of
current smokers in some age groups and these observed differences may
be due to sampling fluctuations. No attempt was made to apply any correc-
tions to these potentially downward biases.

For men, the difference between the annual health service costs of current
and never smokers decreases from £59 in the youngest age group (aged
16–24 years) to £17 in those aged 35–54 years, and increases to £98 in
those aged 75 or older. For women, this difference is largest in the youngest
age group (£182 per annum) and declines through the older age groups.

Defining GP practice profiles and regional data

The proportion of the population currently smoking varies across the
regions of England and Wales. This variation in smoking will generally
reflect the different demographic and socio-economic structures of the
population. Two methods were used to reflect regional differences in
smoking status and the consequent costs to primary care and the health
service more generally. The GHS provides information on the standard
region in which each individual lives. Current smoking rates by gender,
age and region were calculated using the 1990 GHS. For each region the
implications of the different smoking rates in terms of additional health
service use by current smokers relative to never smokers were calculated
for the average practice list (the number of registered patients) of that
region.[17] These figures give the picture of the 'typical' practice in the region.

In reality smoking status is likely to vary more within these large areas
than between them. To capture the effects of different age structures and
economic status in different areas two other practice profiles were constructed for each area in England. The first step was to use the GHS to find
the proportions of the population in different smoking groups by age and
economic status, e.g. employed, unemployed, retired. The results of the

1991 Census for different districts within a region were then used to construct the economic and demographic profiles of two GP practices.

In each region one urban and one rural district were selected. Average list sizes for each region were used.[17] The 1991 Census reports give figures on the numbers of individuals in different 'lifestages', defined by their age, the existence of children in the household and whether the household is headed by a couple. The proportions of the population in each lifestage category and the total number of adult patients were used to predict the average number of current smokers per GP. These numbers were 'adjusted' using district figures on economic status to reflect, for example, that the unemployed are more likely to be current smokers than the employed. Using the predicted number of current smokers for the practice the additional costs were calculated using the methodology described above. Whilst these calculations include an adjustment for some of the important predictors of smoking status, other important characteristics, such as ethnicity, have not been specifically included.

REFERENCES

1. Health Education Authority (1991) *The Smoking Epidemic: Counting the Cost*. HEA. (14 volumes covering each regional health authority)
2. Roberts, J. L. and Graveling, P. A. (1985) *The Big Kill: the Smoking Epidemic in England and Wales*. HEA and BMA.
3. Callum, C., Johnson, K. and Killoran, A. (1992) *The Smoking Epidemic: a Manifesto for Action*. HEA.
4. *The Health of the Nation: a Strategy for England* (1992) Cm 1986. HMSO.
5. Boulton, M. and Williams, A. (1983) 'Health education in the general practice consultation – doctors' advice on diet, alcohol and smoking', *Health Education Journal*, **42**, 57–63.
6. Sanders, D. (1992) *Smoking Cessation Interventions: Is Patient Education Effective?* London School of Hygiene and Tropical Medicine.
7. Russell, M. A. H., Wilson, C., Taylor, C. and Baker, C. D. (1979) 'Effect of general practitioners' advice against smoking', *British Medical Journal*, **2**, 231–35.
8. Foulds, J. (1993) 'Is nicotine replacement therapy effective?', *Addiction*, **88**.
9. Prochaska, J. O., DiClemente, C. C. and Norcross, J. C. (1992) 'In search of how people change – applications to addictive behaviours', *American Psychologist*, **47**, 1102–14.
10. Mason, P., Hunt, P., Raw, M. and Sills, M. (1993) *Helping People Change: a Training Course for Primary Health Care Professionals*. HEA.
11. Hodgson, T. A. (1992) 'Cigarette smoking and lifetime medical expenditure', *Millbank Quarterly*, **70**(1), 81–125.
12. Manning, W. G., Keeler, E. B., Newhouse, J. P., Sloss, E. M. and Wasserman, J. (1989) 'The taxes of sin: do smokers and drinkers pay their way?', *Journal of the American Medical Association*, **261**(11), 1604–9.
13. Treasury (1992) *The Government's Expenditure Plans 1993–4 to 1995–6: Department of Health and Office of Population Censuses and Surveys*, Cm 2212. HMSO.
14. Office of Health Economics (1992) *Compendium of Health Statistics*. 8th edn, OHE.
15. Department of Health (1993) *Health Service Indicators 1990/91*.
16. Jarvis, M. and Jackson, P. (1988) 'Cigar and pipe smoking in Britain – implications for smoking prevalence and cessation', *British Journal of Addiction*, **83**(3), 323–30.
17. Department of Health (1993) *GMS Basic Statistics, England and Wales*. NHS Management Executive, Leeds.